39 Low Sodium Juice Recipes:

Reduce the Amount of Salt You Consume Using Organic Ingredients that Taste Great

By

Joe Correa CSN

COPYRIGHT

© 2017 Live Stronger Faster Inc.

All rights reserved

Reproduction or translation of any part of this work beyond that permitted by section 107 or 108 of the 1976 United States Copyright Act without the permission of the copyright owner is unlawful.

This publication is designed to provide accurate and authoritative information in regard to the subject matter covered. It is sold with the understanding that neither the author nor the publisher is engaged in rendering medical advice. If medical advice or assistance is needed, consult with a doctor. This book is considered a guide and should not be used in any way detrimental to your health. Consult with a physician before starting this nutritional plan to make sure it's right for you.

ACKNOWLEDGEMENTS

This book is dedicated to my friends and family that have had mild or serious illnesses so that you may find a solution and make the necessary changes in your life.

39 Low Sodium Juice Recipes:

Reduce the Amount of Salt You Consume Using Organic Ingredients that Taste Great

By

Joe Correa CSN

CONTENTS

Copyright

Acknowledgements

About The Author

Introduction

39 Low Sodium Juice Recipes: Reduce the Amount of Salt You Consume Using Organic Ingredients that Taste Great

Additional Titles from This Author

ABOUT THE AUTHOR

After years of Research, I honestly believe in the positive effects that proper nutrition can have over the body and mind. My knowledge and experience has helped me live healthier throughout the years and which I have shared with family and friends. The more you know about eating and drinking healthier, the sooner you will want to change your life and eating habits.

Nutrition is a key part in the process of being healthy and living longer so get started today. The first step is the most important and the most significant.

INTRODUCTION

39 Low Sodium Juice Recipes: Reduce the Amount of Salt You Consume Using Organic Ingredients that Taste Great

By Joe Correa CSN

Sodium is a mineral naturally found in foods and one of the essential minerals in the human body. It plays the important role of balancing fluids in the body and regulating muscle contraction. It's often added to some highly processed foods to increase flavor, retain moisture, and extend shelf-life.

However, too much sodium can have devastating effects on the human body and lead to hypertention, kidney disease, cardiovascular disease, and heart attacks. That's why a perfect sodium balance is an extremely important part of every healthy diet.

The main source of sodium in your everyday diet is salt. Unfortunately, most people are not aware of the amounts of salt they consume every day. Some statistics suggest that the average American eats five or even more teaspoons of salt every single day which is about 20 times more than what the body actually needs. This results in holding the excess fluid in the body which creates a significant burden on the heart followed by serious, life-threatening conditions.

Fortunately, this problem can easily be solved through a healthy diet and some small changes that will keep your health and well-being in check. Following a low-sodium diet means reducing the amounts of salt in your everyday meals which can easily be done while cooking. The actual problem lies in buying highly processed foods that often contain some ridiculously high amounts of salt. Make sure to check the nutrition labels of the foods you're buying when you go to the supermarket.

Adopting these healthy habits will reduce fluid accumulation in your body and ease the job of the kidneys which will result in significantly improved overall health.

Being someone who is focused on health and well-being, I have been looking for the best way to clean my body and flush down all the unhealthy substances from my body. This book is a result of that research and personal experience.

This book is a wonderful collection of low-sodium juice recipes that I like to prepare for myself and I am sure you will enjoy.

These juices are a true nutritional treasure that will help your body clean itself and give you a nice boost of vitamins and minerals, while being low-sodium at the same time. Enjoy them all and see the results they have on your health. You deserve it!

39 LOW SODIUM JUICE RECIPES: REDUCE THE AMOUNT OF SALT YOU CONSUME USING ORGANIC INGREDIENTS THAT TASTE GREAT

1. Mango Lime Juice

Ingredients:

1 large mango

1 large lime, peeled

1 large guava, peeled

3 oz of coconut water

Preparation:

Peel the mango and cut into small chunks. Set aside.

Peel the lime and cut lengthwise in half. Set aside.

Wash the guava and cut into chunks. If you are using large fruit, reserve the rest for some other recipe in a refrigerator. Set aside.

Now, process mango, lime, and guava in a juicer. Transfer to serving glasses and stir in the coconut water.

Add few ice cubes and serve immediately.

Enjoy!

Nutritional information per serving: Kcal: 225, Protein: 4.4g, Carbs: 63.9g, Fats: 1.8g

2. Kale Grapefruit Juice

Ingredients:

1 cup of kale, chopped

1 whole grapefruit, peeled

2 cups of grapes

1 cup of watercress, chopped

½ cup of water

Preparation:

Combine kale and watercress in a colander and wash thoroughly. Chop it roughly using hands and set aside.

Wash the grapefruit and cut into chunks. Set aside.

Place the grapes in a colander and wash under cold running water. Set aside.

Now, process grapes, kale, watercress, grapefruit, and grapes in a juicer. Transfer to serving glasses and stir in the water.

Refrigerate for 10 minutes before serving.

Nutritional information per serving: Kcal: 231, Protein: 6.7g, Carbs: 64g, Fats: 1.6g

3. Cabbage Pumpkin Juice

Ingredients:

1 cup of purple cabbage

1 cup of pumpkin, seeded and peeled

1 large orange, peeled

1 large green apple, cored

1 tsp of ginger root

Preparation:

Wash the cabbage thoroughly and torn with hands. Set aside.

Peel the pumpkin and cut in half. Scoop out the seeds using a spoon. Cut one large wedge and peel it. Cut into small chunks and set aside.

Peel the orange and divide into wedges. Set aside.

Wash the apple and remove the core. Cut into bite-sized pieces and set aside.

Peel the ginger root and set aside.

Now, process pumpkin, orange, cabbage, apple, and ginger root in a juicer. Transfer to serving glasses and add few ice cubes.

Refrigerate for 10 minutes before serving.

Nutritional information per serving: Kcal: 228, Protein: 5.4g, Carbs: 69.3g, Fats: 1.5g

4. Strawberry Cranberry Juice

Ingredients:

1 cup of strawberries

1 cup of cranberries

1 small papaya, seeded and peeled

1 large lime, peeled

3 oz of coconut water

Preparation:

Place the strawberries and cranberries in a colander and wash under cold running water. Drain and set aside.

Peel the papaya and cut lengthwise in half. Scoop out the black seeds and flesh using a spoon. Cut into small chunks and set aside.

Peel the lime and cut lengthwise in half. Set aside.

Now, process strawberries, cranberries, papaya, and lime in a juicer. Transfer to serving glasses and stir in the coconut water.

Add some ice, or refrigerate for 10 minutes before serving.

Enjoy!

Nutritional information per serving: Kcal: 153, Protein: 2.6g, Carbs: 50.9g, Fats: 1.8g

5. Radish Mint Juice

Ingredients:

1 medium-sized radish, sliced

1 tbsp of fresh mint, chopped

2 large pears, peeled and seeds removed

1 cup of blueberries, fresh

1 cup of cauliflower, chopped

¼ cup of coconut water, unsweetened

Preparation:

Wash the radish and trim off the green parts. Cut into small pieces and set aside.

Wash the pears and remove the core. Cut into bite-sized pieces and set aside.

Wash the blueberries under cold running water. Drain and set aside.

Trim off the outer leaves of cauliflower. Wash it and cut into small pieces. Reserve the rest in the refrigerator.

Now, process radish, mint, pears, blueberries, and cauliflower in a juicer.

Transfer to serving glasses and stir in the coconut water.

Add some ice and serve.

Nutritional information per serving: Kcal: 297, Protein: 4.9g, Carbs: 97g, Fats: 1.4g

6. Brussels Sprout Leek Juice

Ingredients:

1 cup of Brussels sprouts, chopped

2 large leeks

1 medium-sized fennel bulb, chopped

½ tsp of fresh rosemary

Preparation:

Wash the Brussels sprouts and trim off the outer leaves. Cut into small pieces and set aside.

Wash the leeks and chop into small pieces. Set aside.

Wash the fennel bulb and trim off the wilted outer layers. Cut into small chunks and set aside.

Now, process Brussels sprouts, leeks, and fennel in a juicer. Transfer to serving glasses and sprinkle with finely chopped rosemary. Refrigerate for 10 minutes before serving.

Enjoy!

Nutritional information per serving: Kcal: 165, Protein: 8.5g, Carbs: 50.1g, Fats: 1.3g

7. Cranberry Spinach Juice

Ingredients:

1 cup of cranberries

1 cup of baby spinach, torn

1 cup of turnip greens, chopped

1 whole lemon, peeled

½ cup of pure coconut water

Preparation:

Place the cranberries in a colander and wash under cold running water. Drain and set aside.

Wash the baby spinach thoroughly and torn it with hands.

Wash the turnip greens and roughly chop it using hands. Set aside.

Peel the lemon and cut lengthwise. Set aside.

Now, process cranberries, baby spinach, turnip greens, and lemon in a juicer. Transfer to serving glasses and add pure coconut water.

Add some ice and serve immediately.

Nutritional information per serving: Kcal: 69, Protein: 4.3g, Carbs: 27.6g, Fats: 0.8g

8. Radish Zucchini Juice

Ingredients:

1 small radish, trimmed

1 large zucchini, chopped

1 cup of red leaf lettuce, torn

1 medium-sized sweet potato, peeled

1 tsp of ginger, ground

Preparation:

Wash the radish and trim off the green ends. Chop into small pieces and set aside.

Peel the zucchini and cut it lengthwise in half. Scoop out the seeds and chop into chunks. Set aside.

Peel the sweet potato and place it in a pot of boiling water. Cook until fork-tender and remove from the heat. Drain well and set aside to cool. Chop into small pieces and set aside.

Wash the lettuce thoroughly and torn with hands. Set aside.

Peel the ginger root and set aside.

Now, process radish, zucchini, lettuce, sweet potato, and ginger in a juicer. Transfer to serving glasses and add some water to adjust the thickness, if needed.

Serve immediately.

Nutritional information per serving: Kcal: 67, Protein: 4.3g, Carbs: 18.6g, Fats: 0.8g

9. Cauliflower Leek Juice

Ingredients:

1 cup of broccoli, chopped

1 small cauliflower head

1 large leek

1 cup of fresh kale, torn

1 large green apple, cored

2 oz of water

Preparation:

Trim off the outer leaves of a cauliflower. Cut into bite-sized pieces and set aside.

Wash the leek and chop into small pieces. Set aside.

Wash the broccoli and chop into small pieces. Set aside.

Wash the kale thoroughly under cold running water and torn with hands. Set aside.

Wash the apple and remove the core. Cut into bite-sized pieces and set aside.

Now, process cauliflower, leek, broccoli, kale, and apple in a juicer. Transfer to serving glasses and stir in the water.

Add some ice cubes and serve immediately.

Enjoy!

Nutritional information per serving: Kcal: 233, Protein: 12.7g, Carbs: 65.7g, Fats: 2.3g

10. Banana Zucchini Juice

Ingredients:

1 large Granny Smith's apple, cored

1 large orange, wedged

1 large banana, sliced

1 medium-sized zucchini, sliced

2 oz of water

Preparation:

Wash the apple and remove the core. Cut into bite-sized pieces and set aside.

Peel the orange and divide into wedges. Set aside.

Peel the banana and cut into small chunks. Set aside.

Peel the zucchini and cut in half. Scoop out the seeds and cut into small pieces. Set aside.

Now, process banana, zucchini, apple, and orange in a juicer. Transfer to serving glasses and refrigerate for 10 minutes before serving.

Enjoy!

Nutritional information per serving: Kcal: 296, Protein: 6.5g, Carbs: 86.8g, Fats: 1.7g

11. Apple Cranberry Juice

Ingredients:

1 cup of strawberries, chopped

1 large Granny Smith's apple, cored

1 cup of cranberries

1 large carrot, sliced

1 whole lemon, peeled

1 large orange, peeled and wedged

Preparation:

Wash the apple and remove the core. Cut into bite-sized pieces and set aside.

Place the strawberries and cranberries in a colander and wash under cold running water. Drain and cut in half. Set aside.

Wash the carrot and cut into thick slices. Set aside.

Peel the lemon cut lengthwise in half. Set aside.

Peel the orange and divide into wedges. Set aside.

Now, process apple, cranberries, strawberries, carrots,

lemon, and orange in juicer. Transfer to serving glasses and stir in the water.

Add few ice cubes, or refrigerate for 10 minutes before serving.

Nutritional information per serving: Kcal: 268, Protein: 5.6g, Carbs: 89.1g, Fats: 1.6g

12. Lime Cucumber Juice

Ingredients:

3 large beets, trimmed

1 large lime

1 large cucumber

2 celery stalk, chopped

1 small ginger root knob, 1-inch

2 oz of water

Preparation:

Peel the lime and cut lengthwise in half. Set aside.

Wash the cucumber and cut into thick slices. Set aside.

Wash the beets and trim off the green parts. cut into small pieces and set aside.

Wash the celery and chop into bite-sized pieces. Set aside.

Peel the ginger root knob and set aside.

Now, combine beets, lime, cucumber, celery, and ginger in a juicer and process until juiced. Transfer to serving glasses and stir in the water.

Refrigerate for 10 minutes before serving.

Nutritional information per serving: Kcal: 140, Protein: 6.7g, Carbs: 41.6g, Fats: 0.9g

13. Sweet Orange Honey Juice

Ingredients:

1 large orange, peeled and wedged

1 cup of blackberries

1 large Golden Delicious apple, cored and chopped

1 cup of fresh mint, torn

1 tbsp honey

3 oz coconut water

Preparation:

Peel the orange and divide into wedges. Set aside.

Place the blackberries in a colander and wash under cold running water. Drain and set aside.

Wash the apple and remove the core. Cut into bite-sized pieces and set aside.

Place the mint in a bowl and add one cup of lukewarm water. Let it soak for 15 minutes.

Now, combine blackberries, orange, apple, and mint in a juicer and process until juiced.

Transfer to serving glasses and stir in the coconut water and honey. Add some ice and serve immediately.

Enjoy!

Nutritional information per serving: Kcal: 287, Protein: 5.3g, Carbs: 88.4g, Fats: 1.5g

14. Cucumber Carrot Juice

Ingredients:

1 large cucumber, sliced

1 large carrot, sliced

1 cup of avocado, pitted and chopped

1 cup of pomegranate seeds

¼ tsp of nutmeg

3 oz of water

Preparation:

Wash the cucumber and carrot. Cut into thin slices and set aside.

Peel the avocado and cut in half. Remove the pit and cut into small chunks. Set aside.

Cut the top of the pomegranate fruit using a sharp knife. Slice down to each of the white membranes inside of the fruit. Pop the seeds into a bowl and set aside.

Now, combine cucumber, carrot, avocado, and pomegranate seeds in a juicer and process until juiced.

Transfer to serving glasses and stir in the water and

nutmeg. Add some ice and serve immediately.

Enjoy!

Nutritional information per serving: Kcal: 319, Protein: 7.1g, Carbs: 46.9g, Fats: 23.5g

15. Melon Banana Juice

Ingredients:

1 large Honeydew melon wedge, chopped

1 large banana

2 cups of green grapes

¼ tsp of cinnamon, ground

2 oz of water

Preparation:

Cut the honeydew melon lengthwise in half. Scoop out the seeds using a spoon. Cut one large wedge and peel it. Cut into small chunks and place in a bowl. Wrap the rest of the melon in a plastic foil and refrigerate.

Peel the banana and cut into small chunks. Set aside.

Combine green and red grapes in a colander and wash under cold running water. Drain and set aside.

Now, combine honeydew melon, banana, and grapes in a juicer.

Transfer to serving glasses and stir in the water. Add some ice before serving.

Enjoy!

Nutritional information per serving: Kcal: 374, Protein: 4.4g, Carbs: 105g, Fats: 1.7g

16. Cranberry Apple Juice

Ingredients:

1 cup of cranberries

1 large green apple, cored and chopped

1 cup of strawberries, chopped

1 cup of fresh kale

1 large cucumber

Preparation:

Combine cranberries and strawberries in a colander and wash under cold running water. Drain and cut strawberries in half. Set aside.

Wash the apple and remove the core. Cut into bite-sized pieces and set aside.

Wash the kale thoroughly and drain. Torn with hands and set aside.

Wash the cucumber and cut into thick slices. Set aside.

Now, process cranberries, apple, strawberries, kale, and cucumber. Transfer to serving glasses.

Add some ice cubes before serving.

Enjoy!

Nutritional information per serving: Kcal: 229, Protein: 7.4g, Carbs: 72g, Fats: 1.9g

17. Carrot Grapefruit Juice

Ingredients:

1 large carrot, sliced

1 large grapefruit, chopped

1 cup of mango, chunked

1 large lemon, peeled and halved

1 small pear, cored and chopped

2 oz of water

Preparation:

Wash the carrot and cut into thick slices. Set aside.

Peel the grapefruit and divide into wedges. Set aside.

Wash the mango and cut into chunks. Fill the measuring cup and reserve the rest for some other juice. Set aside.

Peel the lemon and cut lengthwise in half. Set aside.

Wash the pear and remove the core. Cut into bite-sized pieces and set aside.

Now, process carrot, grapefruit, mango, lemon, and pear in a juicer.

Transfer to serving glasses and add stir in the water. Add some ice cubes or refrigerate for 5 minutes before serving.

Enjoy!

Nutritional information per serving: Kcal: 297, Protein: 5.7g, Carbs: 92.7g, Fats: 1.7g

18. Collard Green Apple Juice

Ingredients:

1 cup of collard greens, torn

1 medium-sized apple, cored

1 medium-sized artichoke, chopped

1 cup of green peas

1 cup of carrots, sliced

2 oz of water

Preparation:

Wash the collard greens thoroughly and torn with hands. Set aside.

Wash the apple and cut in half. Remove the core and cut into bite-sized pieces. Set aside.

Using a sharp knife, trim off the outer layers of the artichoke. Wash it and cut into bite-sized pieces. Set aside.

Place the green peas in a colander and wash under cold running water. Drain and set aside.

Wash the carrots and slice into thin slices. Fill the

measuring cup and reserve the rest for some other juice. Set aside.

Now, process artichoke, green peas, collard greens, and carrots in a juicer. Transfer to serving glasses and refrigerate for 5 minutes before serving.

Nutritional information per serving: Kcal: 250, Protein: 16.2g, Carbs: 74.9g, Fats: 1.7g

19. Apple Lettuce Juice

Ingredients:

1 large apple, cored

1 cup of red leaf lettuce, torn

1 cup of green beans, chopped

1 cup of fresh kale, torn

1 large lime, peeled

1 large red bell pepper, chopped

1 small ginger root knob, 1-inch

3 oz of water

Preparation:

Wash the apple and remove the core. Cut into bite-sized pieces and set aside.

Combine kale and red leaf lettuce in a colander and wash thoroughly under cold running water. Torn with hands and set aside.

Wash the green beans and chop into bite-sized pieces. Set aside.

Peel the lime and cut lengthwise in half. Set aside.

Wash the red bell pepper and cut in half. Remove the seeds and chop into small pieces. Set aside.

Peel the ginger root knob and set aside.

Now, process apple, red leaf lettuce, green beans, kale, lime, red bell pepper, and ginger root in a juicer.

Transfer to serving glasses and stir in the water. Add some ice and serve immediately.

Nutritional information per serving: Kcal: 194, Protein: 7.1g, Carbs: 52.9g, Fats: 1.7g

20. Celery Carrot Juice

Ingredients:

3 large carrots, sliced

1 large cucumber, sliced

2 cups of celery, chopped

1 cup of sweet potatoes, cubed

1 small ginger root knob, 1-inch

Preparation:

Wash the carrots and cucumber. Cut into thick slices and set aside.

Wash the celery and cut into small pieces. Set aside.

Peel the sweet potato and cut into cubes. Fill the measuring cup and reserve the rest for some other juice. Set aside.

Peel the ginger knob and set aside.

Now, process carrots, cucumber, celery, potatoes, and ginger in a juicer.

Transfer to serving glasses and refrigerate for 5 minutes before serving.

Enjoy!

Nutritional information per serving: Kcal: 228, Protein: 7.6g, Carbs: 65.4g, Fats: 1.3g

21. Squash Pomegranate Juice

Ingredients:

1 cup of pomegranate seeds

1 whole lemon, peeled

2 cups of butternut squash, chopped

1 large orange, peeled and wedged

1 cup of celery, chopped

2 oz of water

Preparation:

Cut the top of the pomegranate fruit using a sharp knife. Slice down to each of the white membranes inside of the fruit. Pop the seeds into a medium bowl.

Peel the lemon and orange. Divide orange into wedges and cut lemon lengthwise in half. Set aside.

Peel the butternut squash and remove the seeds using a spoon. Cut into small cubes and reserve the rest of the squash for some other recipe. Wrap in a plastic foil and refrigerate.

Wash the celery and chop into small pieces. Set aside.

Now, combine pomegranate seeds, lemon, butternut squash, orange, and celery in a juicer and process until juiced.

Transfer to serving glasses and stir in the water. Add few ice cubes and serve immediately.

Enjoy!

Nutritional information per serving: Kcal: 251, Protein: 7.3g, Carbs: 79g, Fats: 1.8g

22. Cucumber Basil Juice

Ingredients:

1 large cucumber, sliced

1 cup of fresh basil, torn

3 cups of collard greens, torn

2 large carrots, sliced

1 medium-sized sweet potato, cubed

Preparation:

Wash the cucumber and carrots. Cut into thin slices and set aside.

Combine basil and collard greens in a colander. Wash under cold running water and drain. Torn with hands and set aside.

Peel the sweet potato and chop into cubes. Set aside.

Now, process cucumber, basil, collard greens, carrots, and sweet potato in a juicer. Transfer to serving glasses and refrigerate for 10 minutes or add some ice and serve immediately.

Nutritional information per serving: Kcal: 201, Protein: 9.3g, Carbs: 57.3g, Fats: 1.5g

23. Cauliflower Lime Juice

Ingredients:

1 cup of cauliflower, chopped

1 large lime, peeled

2 medium-sized tomatoes

1 large red bell pepper, chopped

3 oz of water

1 tsp of fresh rosemary, finely chopped

Preparation:

Trim off the outer leaves of cauliflower. Wash it and cut into small pieces. Reserve the rest in the refrigerator.

Peel the lime and cut lengthwise in half. Set aside.

Wash the tomatoes and place them in a bowl. Cut into quarters and reserve the juice while cutting. Set aside.

Wash the bell pepper and cut in half. Remove the seeds and chop into small slices. Set aside.

Now, combine cauliflower, lime, tomatoes, and red bell pepper in a juicer and process until juiced.

Transfer to serving glasses and stir in the reserved tomato juice and water. Sprinkle with fresh rosemary for some extra taste.

Refrigerate for 5 minutes before serving.

Enjoy!

Nutritional information per serving: Kcal: 98, Protein: 6g, Carbs: 28.5g, Fats: 1.3g

24. Swiss Chard Cucumber Juice

Ingredients:

1 cup of Swiss chard, torn

1 cup of cucumber, sliced

2 cups of parsnips, chopped

1 large green bell pepper, chopped

1 ginger root knob, 1-inch

2 oz of water

Preparation:

Wash the Swiss chard thoroughly and torn with hands. Set aside.

Wash the cucumber and cut into thin slices. Fill the measuring cup and reserve the rest for later.

Peel the ginger and set aside.

Now, process Swiss chard, cucumber, parsnips, bell pepper, and ginger knob in a juicer.

Transfer to serving glasses and stir in the water.

Add some ice and serve immediately.

Enjoy!

Nutritional information per serving: Kcal: 219, Protein: 7.3g, Carbs: 68.8g, Fats: 1.5g

25. Grapefruit Cucumber Juice

Ingredients:

1 large grapefruit, peeled and wedged

1 large cucumber, sliced

1 cup of papaya, chopped

1 small green apple, cored and chopped

2 oz of coconut water

Preparation:

Peel the grapefruit and divide into wedges. Set aside.

Wash the cucumber and cut into thick slices. Set aside.

Peel the papaya and cut lengthwise in half. Scoop out the black seeds and flesh using a spoon. Cut into small chunks and fill the measuring cup. Reserve the rest for some other juice. Set aside.

Wash the apple and remove the core. Cut into bite-sized pieces and set aside.

Now, process grapefruit, cucumber, papaya, and apple in a juicer. Transfer to serving glasses and stir in the coconut water.

Add few ice cubes and serve immediately.

Nutritional information per serving: Kcal: 246, Protein: 5.1g, Carbs: 72.4g, Fats: 1.3g

26. Carrot Orange Juice

Ingredients:

1 large carrot, sliced

1 large orange, peeled and wedged

1 cup of cherries, halved and pitted

1 small apple, cored

1 whole lemon, peeled

2 oz of water

Preparation:

Wash the carrot and cut into thick slices. Set aside.

Peel the orange and lemon. Divide orange into wedges and cut lemon lengthwise in half. Set aside.

Wash the cherries thoroughly and cut into halves. Remove the pits and set aside.

Wash the apple and remove the core. Cut into bite-sized pieces and set aside.

Now, combine carrot, orange, lemon, cherries, and apple in a juicer and process until juiced. Transfer to serving glasses and add some ice before serving.

Enjoy!

Nutritional information per serving: Kcal: 253, Protein: 5.3g, Carbs: 78.2g, Fats: 1.1g

27. Pumpkin Pineapple Juice

Ingredients:

1 cup of pineapple chunks

1 medium-sized zucchini

1 cup of pumpkin, chopped

1 cup of apricot, chopped

1 medium-sized apple, cored

2 oz of water

Preparation:

Cut the top of a pineapple and peel it using a sharp knife. Cut into small chunks. Reserve the rest of the pineapple in a refrigerator.

Peel the zucchini and cut in half. Scoop out the seeds and cut into cubes. Set aside. Peel the pumpkin and cut in half. Scoop out the seeds using a spoon. Cut one large wedge and peel it. Cut into small chunks and set aside. Reserve the rest for later.

Wash the apricots and cut in half. Remove the pits and cut into pieces. Fill the measuring cup and reserve the rest for some other juice. Set aside.

Wash the apple and remove the core. Cut into bite-sized pieces and set aside.

Now, process pineapple, zucchini, pumpkin, apricots, and apple in a juicer.

Transfer to serving glasses and stir in the water. Add some ice and serve immediately.

Nutritional information per serving: Kcal: 272, Protein: 7.2g, Carbs: 76.6g, Fats: 1.8g

28. Mint Orange Juice

Ingredients:

1 cup of fresh mint, chopped

1 large orange, peeled

1 large green apple, cored

1 handful of fresh spinach, torn

3 oz of water

Preparation:

Combine mint and spinach in a colander and wash thoroughly under cold running water. Drain and torn with hands.

Peel the orange and divide into wedges. Set aside.

Wash the apple and remove the core. Cut into bite-sized pieces and set aside.

Now, combine apple, orange, mint, and spinach in a juicer and process until juiced. Transfer to serving glasses and then stir in the water.

Add some ice before serving and enjoy!

Nutritional information per serving: Kcal: 178, Protein: 4.4g, Carbs: 54.5g, Fats: 0.9g

29. Cantaloupe Basil Juice

Ingredients:

1 cup of cantaloupe, chopped

1 cup of fresh basil, chopped

1 cup of cauliflower, chopped

1 cup of fresh kale, chopped

1 medium-sized cucumber, sliced

Preparation:

Cut the cantaloupe in half. Scoop out the seeds and flesh. Cut two wedges and peel them. Chop into chunks and set aside. Reserve the rest of the cantaloupe in a refrigerator.

Combine basil and kale in a colander under cold running water. Drain and roughly chop it.

Trim off the outer leaves of cauliflower. Wash it and cut into small pieces. Fill the measuring cup and reserve the rest in the refrigerator.

Wash the cucumber and cut into thick pieces. set aside.

Now, combine cantaloupe, basil, cauliflower, kale, and cucumber in a juicer and process until juiced. Transfer to serving glasses and add few ice cubes before serving.

Enjoy!

Nutritional information per serving: Kcal: 132, Protein: 8.9g, Carbs: 35.4g, Fats: 1.7g

30. Lime Orange Juice

Ingredients:

1 cup of avocado, chopped

1 large lime, peeled

1 large orange, peeled

1 large cucumber, sliced

2 oz of water

Preparation:

Peel the lime and cut lengthwise in half. Set aside.

Peel the orange and divide into wedges. Set aside.

Peel the avocado and cut in half. Remove the pit and cut into small chunks. Fill the measuring cup and reserve the rest for some other juice.

Wash the cucumber and cut into thick slices. Set aside.

Now, combine lime, orange, avocado, and cucumber in a juicer and process until juiced. Transfer to serving glasses and stir in the water.

Add some ice and serve immediately.

Nutritional information per serving: Kcal: 132, Protein: 8.9g, Carbs: 35.4g, Fats: 1.7g

31. Kiwi Lemon Juice

Ingredients:

2 large kiwis, peeled

1 large lemon, peeled

1 cup of pineapple chunks

1 large carrot

1 large yellow apple, cored

1 tbsp of liquid honey

Preparation:

Peel the kiwis and lemon. Cut lengthwise in half and set aside.

Cut the top of a pineapple and peel it using a sharp knife. Cut into small chunks and fill the measuring cup. Reserve the rest of the pineapple in a refrigerator.

Wash the carrot and cut into thick slices. Set aside.

Wash the apple and remove the core. Cut into bite-sized pieces and set aside.

Now, process kiwis, lemon, pineapple, carrot, and apple in a juicer. Transfer to serving glasses and stir in the honey.

Optionally, add some vanilla extract for some extra taste.

Add some ice before serving.

Nutritional information per serving: Kcal: 132, Protein: 8.9g, Carbs: 35.4g, Fats: 1.7g

32. Spinach Orange Juice

Ingredients:

1 cup of spinach, torn

1 large orange, peeled

1 cup of butternut squash, cubed

1 large cucumber

1 ginger root slice, 1-inch

Preparation:

Wash the spinach thoroughly under cold running water. Drain and torn with hands. Set aside.

Peel the orange and divide into wedges. Set aside.

Peel the butternut squash and remove the seeds using a spoon. Cut into small cubes and reserve the rest of the squash for some other recipe. Wrap in a plastic foil and refrigerate.

Wash the cucumber and cut into thick slices. Set aside.

Peel the ginger root slice and set aside.

Now, combine spinach, orange, squash, cucumber, and ginger slice in a juicer and process until juiced.

Add some ice and water if necessary and serve immediately.

Enjoy!

Nutritional information per serving: Kcal: 209, Protein: 14.8g, Carbs: 61.6g, Fats: 2.1g

33. Lime Orange Juice

Ingredients:

1 large lime, peeled

2 large oranges, peeled

2 large lemons, peeled

1 cup of fresh mint, torn

¼ tsp of pure peppermint extract

Preparation:

Peel the lime and lemons. Cut lengthwise in half and set aside.

Peel the orange and divide into wedges. Set aside.

Place the mint in a colander and wash thoroughly under cold running water. Drain and torn with hands. Set aside.

Now, combine lime, lemons, orange, and mint in a juicer and process until juiced. Transfer to a serving glass and stir in the peppermint extract.

Add some water if needed.

Refrigerate for 10 minutes before serving.

Nutritional information per serving: Kcal: 178, Protein: 5.8g, Carbs: 61.5g, Fats: 1.1g

34. Lettuce Lemon Juice

Ingredients:

1 cup of red leaf lettuce, torn

1 large lemon, peeled

4 large carrots, sliced

1 large red apple, cored

Preparation:

Wash the lettuce thoroughly under cold running water. Torn with hands and set aside.

Peel the lemon and cut lengthwise in half. Set aside.

Wash the carrots and cut into thick slices. Set aside.

Wash the apple and remove the core. Cut into bite-sized pieces and set aside.

Now, process lettuce, lemon, carrots, and apple in a juicer. Transfer to serving glasses and add some ice before serving.

Enjoy!

Nutritional information per serving: Kcal: 231, Protein: 4.4g, Carbs: 70g, Fats: 1.4g

35. Leek Broccoli Juice

Ingredients:

3 large leeks, chopped

1 cup of broccoli, chopped

3 cups of kale, chopped

1 large cucumber

1 small ginger root slice, 1-inch

Preparation:

Wash the leeks and cut into small pieces. Set aside.

Wash the broccoli and cut into bite-sized pieces. Fill the measuring cup and reserve the rest for some other juice.

Wash the kale thoroughly under cold running water using a colander. Drain and torn roughly chop it. Set aside.

Wash the cucumber and cut into thick slices. Set aside.

Peel the ginger root slice and set aside.

Now, process leeks, broccoli, kale, cucumber and ginger in a juicer.

Transfer to serving glasses and refrigerate for 10 minutes

before serving.

Nutritional information per serving: Kcal: 275, Protein: 17.2g, Carbs: 72.7g, Fats: 3.3g

36. Grape Watermelon Juice

Ingredients:

1 cup of green grapes

1 cup of watermelon, seeded and chopped

1 cup of mango, chopped

1 large Fuji apple, cored

2 oz of water

Preparation:

Wash the green grapes using a colander and set aside.

Cut the watermelon lengthwise. For one cup, you will need about 1 large wedge. Peel and cut into chunks. Remove the seeds and set aside. Reserve the rest for some other juice.

Wash the mango and cut into chunks. Set aside.

Wash the apple and remove the core. Cut into bite-sized pieces and set aside.

Now, combine grapes, watermelon, mango, and apple in a juicer and process until juiced.

Transfer to serving glasses and stir in the water. Add few

ice cubes or refrigerate before serving.

Enjoy!

Nutritional information per serving: Kcal: 288, Protein: 3.7g, Carbs: 80g, Fats: 1.5g

37. Pumpkin Pie Juice

Ingredients:

1 cup of pumpkin, chopped

1 cup of sweet potato, chopped

1 medium-sized carrot, sliced

1 medium-sized cucumber, sliced

1 medium-sized zucchini, chopped

¼ tsp of ginger, ground

Preparation:

Peel the pumpkin and cut in half. Scoop out the seeds using a spoon. Cut one large wedge and peel it. Cut into small chunks and fill the measuring cup. Reserve the rest for later.

Peel the sweet potato and cut into small chunks. Place in a potof boiling water and cook for 10 minutes. Remove from the heat and drain. Set aside to cool completely.

Wash the carrot and cut into thick slices. Set aside.

Peel the zucchini and cut in half. Scrape out the seeds using a spoon. Cut into bite-sized pieces and set aside.

Wash the cucumber and cut into thick slices. Set aside.

Now, combine pumpkin, cooked potato, carrot, cucumber, and zucchini in a juicer and process until juiced.

Transfer to serving glasses and stir in the ginger.

Add some ice and serve.

Nutritional information per serving: Kcal: 214, Protein: 8.3g, Carbs: 58.6g, Fats: 1.3g

38. Guava Orange Juice

Ingredients:

1 large guava, chopped

1 large orange, peeled

1 large lime, peeled

1 medium-sized apple, cored

3 oz of water

Preparation:

Peel and wash the guava. Cut into small chunks and set aside.

Peel the orange and divide into wedges. Set aside.

Peel the lime and cut lengthwise in half. Set aside.

Wash the apple and remove the core. Cut into bite-sized pieces and set aside.

Now, combine guava, orange, lime, and apple in a juicer and process until juiced.

Transfer to a serving glass and stir in the water. Add some ice and serve immediately.

Nutritional information per serving: Kcal: 163, Protein: 3.5g, Carbs: 49.7g, Fats: 1g

39. Apple Orange Juice

Ingredients:

1 medium-sized Red Delicious apple, cored and chopped

1 large orange, peeled and wedged

2 large peaches, pitted and chopped

1 ginger root slice, peeled

1 tbsp of honey, raw

2 oz of water

Preparation:

Wash the apple and remove the core. Cut into bite-sized pieces and set aside.

Peel the orange and divide into wedges. Set aside.

Wash the peaches and cut in half. Remove the pits and cut into small pieces.

Peel the ginger root slice and set aside.

Now, process peaches, apple, orange, and ginger in a juicer. Transfer to serving glasses and stir in the honey and water.

Add a few ice cubes before serving and enjoy!

Nutritional information per serving: Kcal: 323, Protein: 5.6g, Carbs: 97.4g, Fats: 1.4g

ADDITIONAL TITLES FROM THIS AUTHOR

70 Effective Meal Recipes to Prevent and Solve Being Overweight: Burn Fat Fast by Using Proper Dieting and Smart Nutrition

By Joe Correa CSN

48 Acne Solving Meal Recipes: The Fast and Natural Path to Fixing Your Acne Problems in Less Than 10 Days!

By Joe Correa CSN

41 Alzheimer's Preventing Meal Recipes: Reduce or Eliminate Your Alzheimer's Condition in 30 Days or Less!

By Joe Correa CSN

70 Effective Breast Cancer Meal Recipes: Prevent and Fight Breast Cancer with Smart Nutrition and Powerful Foods

By Joe Correa CSN

www.ingramcontent.com/pod-product-compliance
Lightning Source LLC
Chambersburg PA
CBHW030301030426
42336CB00009B/473